IT'S YOUR DECISION

A GUIDE TO HELP YOU MAKE INFORMED MEDICAL DECISIONS

CAMILLE M. RENELLA

AuthorHouse™
1663 Liberty Drive
Bloomington, IN 47403
www.authorhouse.com
Phone: 1 (800) 839-8640

Published by AuthorHouse 04/07/2020

ISBN: 978-1-7283-1921-6 (sc)
ISBN: 978-1-7283-1920-9 (e)

Print information available on the last page.

authorHOUSE®

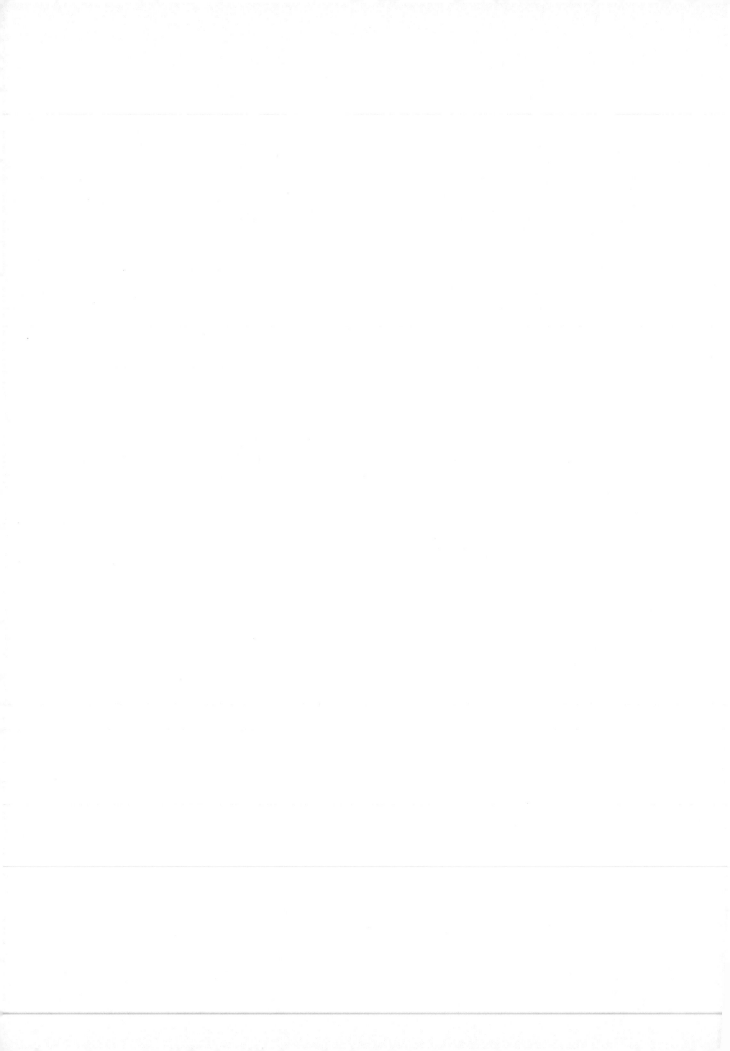

IT'S YOUR DECISION

Getting the information you need to make informed medical decisions that reflect your values, lifestyle, wishes and goals.

Medical Treatment Decisions are made after considering the Medical Indications, Quality of Life, your values and preferences and other circumstances.

Your Healthcare Team includes the Attending Physician, treating physicians, primary nurse, social worker, case manager and other healthcare professionals assigned to care for you.

Contents

ABOUT THE AUTHOR

Camille M. Renella is a veteran clinician and former Associate Faculty Member of The MacLean Center for Clinical Medical Ethics at the University of Chicago. Camille completed the Post Doctorate Fellowship in Clinical Medical Ethics at the University of Chicago Pritzker School of Medicine and served as Chief Ethicist in Patient Services at The University of Chicago Hospitals and The University of Chicago Children's Hospital for ten years. Camille has an extensive clinical background in adult, child and home health nursing, as well as Nursing Administration and Multidisciplinary staff education. Camille continues to integrate her background in medicine, law and clinical medical ethics as President of her National Consulting Firm, C.M. RENELLA & ASSOCIATES and currently, as Executive Director of Healthcare Competency Program Specialists, LLC.

Throughout her career Camille participated in Clinical Outreach Programs in San Juan, Puerto Rico and in a Capitol Hill, Washington DC nation-wide initiative. Camille provided presentations at local, national and international conferences, was an Ambassador to Eastern European countries of Hungary, Czechoslovakia and Poland where she participated in ethics discussions with members of the countries' medical associations, was an Associate of the American Bar Association (ABA), ABA Board Member – New Member Committee – Health Law Division, also an ABA Associate Membership Chair – New Member Committee of the Health Law Division, was a member of the American Society of Law, Medicine, and Ethics Hastings Center, People to People Ambassador Program, U. S. Ambassador for Medical Ethics, American Association of Legal Nurse Consultants (AALNC), member of the American Association of Legal Nurse Consultants (AALNC) Chicago Chapter, Vice President & Program Chairman of the Women's Council of the Brain Research Foundation at the University of Chicago and is an Institute of Medicine Chicago (IOMC) fellow. Camille also served as a member of the Harrington Institute of Design, Chicago Alumni Board of Directors.

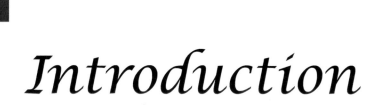

Introduction

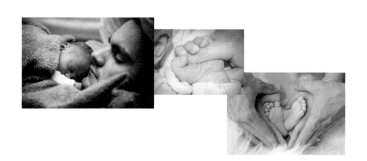

"Decisions are the frequent fabric
of our daily design."

~ Don Yaeger

IT'S YOUR DECISION

The medical decision-making process emphasizes patient-centered care as a method of care that relies upon effective communication and a feeling of partnership between Doctor, healthcare provider and patient to improve patient care outcomes and satisfaction, to lessen patient symptoms, and to reduce unnecessary costs.

Doctors and healthcare providers are able to help you become more engaged in your medical treatment decisions and active in the management of your diseases. You should also feel more satisfied with the care you are receiving. This is all achieved while reducing the need for expensive prescriptions, testing, referrals, and hospitalizations. It is a low-tech humanistic approach to medicine with the option of using high tech medicine when necessary, but not as a substitute for the fundamental connection between you and your doctor/healthcare provider. (from Patient-Centered Care: What It Means and How to Get There - James Rickert - January 24, 2012)

Making your desires known by completing this guide, provides you with the assurance that your wishes will be honored and offers your doctor/healthcare provider a clear guide to follow for your medical care.

As we live our life, we make choices. The same is true for making choices about different kinds of medical care. Without sharing your thoughts, your family and your doctor would have to guess what kind of medical care you would want. No guidance would result in a great burden for them. It is also possible you may not receive the care you would want for yourself.

How Do You Make Decisions? As you begin to think about the care you want now and at the end of your life, remember that the reason to make INFORMED DECISIONS is so you receive care that makes you most comfortable. These kinds of individual decisions are based on who you are, your position in your family, your religious beliefs, your ethnic background and traditions, among others. These factors are deeply ingrained in us, and have a powerful influence on all decisions we make. Decisions about your medical care, including how you want to die are no different, which is why we rely on our values or the principles that make us who we are, in order to make the most important decisions of our life.

What are Values? Values are ideals that guide or qualify your personal conduct. Like morals, they help you distinguish what is right from what is wrong and inform you on how you can conduct your life in a meaningful way.

But naming our core values and how we prioritize them can sometimes be a challenge. Although our actions are grounded in core personal values, it still may be difficult to set out a "cookbook" for resolving concerns based on these values. For example,_____in one case,_____in another_____.

Consider this…there are different kinds of Values…**Personal Values** which define you as an individual. Principles such as honesty, reliability and trust determine how you face the world and relate to people. **Cultural Values** define your connection to people with similar backgrounds and help you remain connected to your cultural roots. **Social Values** define how you relate to others in social situations including those involving family, friends and co-workers. **Work Values** define how you relate to your coworkers & clients and guide your behavior in professional contexts.

So, to make informed, medical decisions consider your values. Think about your daily routine. What do you seem to choose more in your life and what do you seem to avoid? Examine past decisions, remember the reason behind an important or difficult decision you made. Think about others who have influenced your life. During the course of our lives, usually without realizing it, we may take on the values and beliefs of those around us as we watch them address the circumstances of their lives. Think of your value system as a set of principles that evolves over time. As we gain life experience, we also gain a clearer understanding of who we are and what we stand for as a person. Now, review the list of Sample Values (see Appendix) and select YOUR personal values. *Add others if they are not listed.*

PERSONAL VALUES – For Example "I value_____" such things as hard work, independence, positive attitude, practicality, privacy, family closeness, competitiveness, appearance, authority-control over activities, competition, physical work, power-having influence and the ability to act on it, knowledge, leadership, personal development, quality relationships, self-respect, order, serenity, self-reliance, etc. (see Appendix for a list of more value examples).

Now make a list of 20 of your personal values. Remember, although you may realize the impact your values have on your everyday decisions, you may not always realize the way they influence how you make medical decisions.

How may your values influence how you make medical decisions? For example: Does the quality of every day matter to you most or do you want to live as long as possible? Are there limits to how much treatment you might want or how much money you are willing to spend or do you value life at any cost? A member of your family may be asked you want to be placed on a breathing machine / ventilator if you stopped breathing. If you had a lung disease that was only going to get worse what would you want the benefit of treatment to be? What if it was clear that you would never be able to live without the machine? Would that change your decision about starting it? Do you feel the use of a ventilator prolongs life or prolongs death? What if you were on a ventilator for two weeks and it looked like you would never recover enough to breathe on your own? Should it be discontinued? What if two weeks or two years passed? When and under what circumstances would you want to discontinue life support?

Now identify 10 values from your list of 20 that are the **most important** guiding principles in your life and rank them according to their importance (#1 being the most important and #10 the least important).

1. _____

2. _____

3. _____

4. _____

5. _____

6. _____

7. _____

8. _____

9. _____

10. _____

From your list, what is the value or values you would absolutely not want to live without?

1. _____   4. _____

2. _____   5. _____

3. _____   6. _____

Now discuss your values and order of their importance with: (3 names, relationship of each, date you discussed these values with each person you chose).

Name	Relationship	Discussion Date
1._____	_____	_____
2._____	_____	_____
3._____	_____	_____

Discuss your values and order of their importance with your doctor(s) and/or healthcare provider(s). Include their names and date of each discussion.

MD/HC Provider Name	Discussion Date
1._____	_____
2._____	_____
3._____	_____

Congratulations for having the foresight and the courage to honor yourself enough to make your informed medical wishes known. There is no better gift to give yourself and to your loved ones. When you are done, you will have the sense of security that comes from knowing you have thought through this decision-making process.

Making your informed medical desires known provides you with the assurance that your wishes will be honored and offers your healthcare providers a clear guide to follow.

Again, remember as we live our life, we make choices – the same is true for making choices about different kinds of medical care. Without sharing your thoughts, your family and your doctor would have to guess what kind of medical care you would want. No guidance would result in a great burden for them. It is also possible you may not receive the care you would want for yourself.

Complete this form, It's Your Decision, during and after you meet with your healthcare provider regarding your diagnosis in order to save time and money, stay focused and maintain effective communication in order for them to respect your informed medical decisions and to assure they ultimately provide you with Optimal Patient-Centered Care……Care based on YOUR values, YOUR wishes and YOUR understanding.

Name	Relation	Contact Info
_____	_____	_____
_____	_____	_____
_____	_____	_____
_____	_____	_____
_____	_____	_____

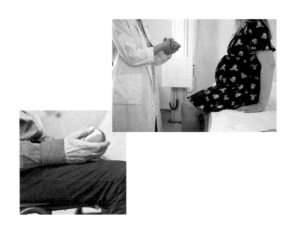

Medical History

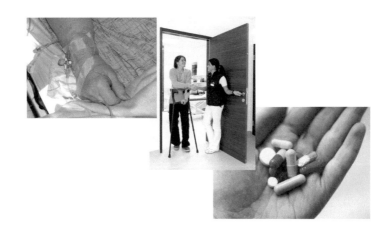

MEDICAL HISTORY

(Patient) Your Name:

Date:

Current Medical Condition or Disease:

Additional Medical Conditions and Diseases:

_____

_____

_____

_____

_____

_____

_____

My Healthcare Team Members:

_____ MD/Nurse Practitioner (NP)

_____ Primary RN

_____ Case Manager

_____ Social Worker

_____ Physical Therapist

_____ Occupational Therapist

_____

_____

_____

_____

Notes:

"Deciding what not to do is as important as deciding what to do."

~ Steve Jobs

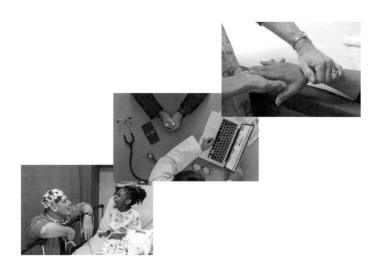

Healthcare Team Meeting

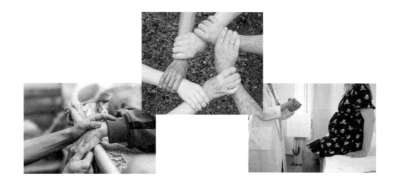

Whenever you receive a medical diagnosis,
you can request a meeting with all the healthcare team members
who will be caring for you throughout the disease and disease treatment process.
Ask to meet with the entire team together at least once, in order for
everyone to share the same information and treatment goals (continuity of care).
Keep a record here, of those team members, for continuous referral throughout
the disease and disease treatment process.

It is also helpful to bring a trusted family member and/or friend to the meeting
in order for them to write the answers to questions listed here. That way you can
listen to the answers and refer to this written documentation when you
are home and later on throughout your decision-making process.

Thought beyond emotions makes better decision-making.

MEETING WITH YOUR DOCTOR AND/OR OTHER HEALTHCARE TEAM MEMBERS

Date: _____ Time: _____

Healthcare Team Participants:

_____ MD/Nurse Practitioner (NP)

_____ RN

_____ Case Manager

_____ Social Worker

_____ Physical Therapist

_____ Occupational Therapist

_____

_____

_____

_____

_____

Family Members and / or Selected Others Attending the Meeting or Doctor's Visit with you:

_____   _____

_____   _____

YOUR CURRENT MEDICAL CONDITION / DISEASE:

Make sure you learn more about this medical condition / disease. You may request pictures, websites, videos, whatever it takes to help you understand the condition/disease and all proposed treatment options.

Ask the following questions to understand the recommended treatment and treatment options:

- What is the **goal** of the **recommended** treatment?

- What are the **benefits** of the **recommended** treatment?

- What are the **risks** of the **recommended** treatment?

- How will the recommended treatment make me feel during treatment administration? What will I need to do to participate in this treatment? (Burdens of Treatment – see Appendix for examples)

- What is the prognosis or expected outcome **with** the recommended treatment?

- What is the prognosis or expected outcome **without** the recommended treatment?

What are my treatment options?

1. _____

2. _____

3. _____

TREATMENT OPTION # 1 -

- What are the **benefits** of treatment option # 1?

- What are the **risks** of treatment option # 1?

- How will this treatment make me feel during treatment administration? What will I need to do to participate in this treatment? (Burdens of Treatment – see Appendix for examples)

- What is the **prognosis** or **expected outcome** with treatment option # 1?

TREATMENT OPTION # 2 -

- What are the **benefits** of treatment option # 2?

- What are the **risks** of treatment option # 2?

- How will this treatment make me feel during treatment administration? What will I need to do to participate in this treatment? (Burdens of Treatment – see Appendix for examples)

- What is the **prognosis** or **expected outcome** with treatment option # 2?

TREATMENT OPTION # 3 -

- What are the **benefits** of treatment option # 3?

- What are the **risks** of treatment option # 3?

- How will this treatment make me feel during treatment administration? What will I need to do to participate in this treatment? (Burdens of Treatment – see Appendix for examples)

- What is the **prognosis** or **expected outcome** with treatment option # 3?

- What are the risks, benefits, burdens and prognosis or expected outcome of **NO treatment?**

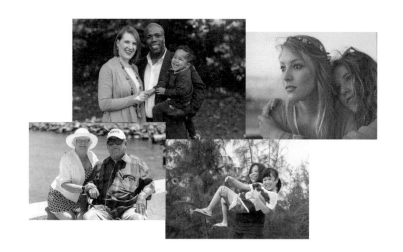

At Home After the Meeting

What are YOUR PREFERENCES?

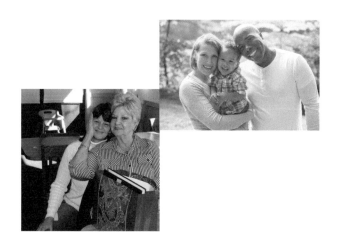

AT HOME AFTER THE MEETING – What are YOUR PREFERENCES?

Think about and then talk about the following with your family:

- Given all the risks, benefits and burdens of all the options you listed above in the previous (purple) section, what treatment option do **you think** you may want?

- Why would you choose this treatment option (consider your values)?

- Why NOT choose the other treatment options (refer again to your values)?

- Do you feel you have enough information to make your decisions?

 List your additional questions here.

 _____
 _____
 _____
 _____

- Do you understand what all treatment options mean **for you**?

- Can you repeat and clearly explain your understanding of each of the risks, burdens, benefits and prognosis (treatment outcome) of each of the options, including the recommended treatment option and the option of NO treatment?

What are the **values** (see list of **examples** in Appendix you considered in making your decision(s)? Start with the one that is most important to you:

1. _____

2. _____

3. _____

4. _____

5. _____

- Are your decisions voluntary and not made under pressure from MD, Family, etc.?

- If, at any point, there is ANY doubt about your capacity to make informed medical treatment decisions for yourself a psychological evaluation may be needed to help determine your capacity to make difficult, complex decisions. That decision making capacity should be formally established and documented in your medical record.

- If, at any time, you demonstrate the lack of understanding, **who will make these medical decisions for you?** Your surrogate is required to make these medical treatment decisions BASED ON YOUR VALUES, whether or not your surrogate agrees with your decisions. **So, make sure you discuss your wishes with your appointed surrogate while you have the mental capacity to do so.**

YOUR QUALITY OF LIFE

- Describe your quality of life NOW.

- What quality of life during and after treatment do you think you would be willing to accept?

- Is your quality of life "less than minimal?"

- * What level of "quality" IS acceptable to YOU?

- * What level of "quality" IS NOT acceptable to you?

At any point in your care consider at what point do you think you would want to stop treatment focused on curing your disease and *quantity* of life and focus instead on *quality* of life and comfort care? Make sure you complete a **Living Will and/or Durable Power of Attorney for Healthcare** to reflect YOUR wishes and discuss your decisions with your family members/selected others, **especially** when you are healthy and not in decision-making crisis. **Make sure your attending MD has a copy of the completed document(s) to include in your medical record. Your doctor and/or a medical ethics consultant can help you with this process as well as completion of your Advance Directives. Just ask one of your healthcare team members for guidance.**

_____

_____

_____

_____

_____

Notes:

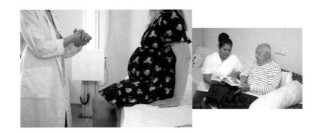

Additional Circumstances

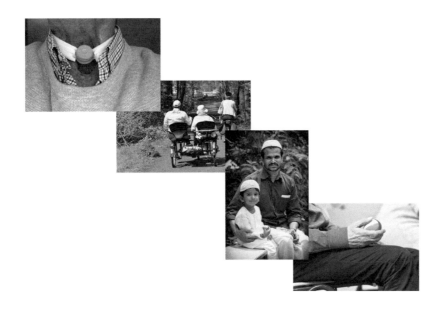

ADDITIONAL CIRCUMSTANCES that may impact your treatment decisions:

Can other circumstances, such as social, legal, economic and institutional circumstances influence these medical decisions?

Yes   _____

No   _____

Maybe _____

Which circumstances and how do they affect your treatment decisions, i.e., inability to pay for treatment; inadequate social support, etc.?

1. _____

_____
_____
_____
_____

2. _____

_____
_____
_____
_____

3. _____

_____
_____
_____

4. _____

_____
_____
_____

5. _____

_____
_____
_____
_____

Additional thoughts, questions for healthcare team and/or specific healthcare team members:

_____

_____

_____

_____

_____

_____

_____

_____

_____

_____

_____

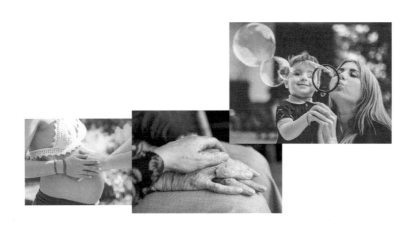

Now...

*Put the Answers
to All the Questions
Together*

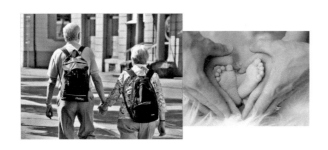

Put the answers to ALL the questions TOGETHER, those listed above + any others you want to add, in order for you to make INFORMED medical treatment decisions that are right for you.
Remember, once you make a treatment decision, you are free to change your mind at any time.

Enter your thoughts and / or decision here:

Be sure to share your wishes, preferences and decision(s) based on your values, with your family, selected others, Attending MD, NP and other members of your Primary Healthcare Team.

I shared my thoughts and/or decisions with:

Name	**Relation**	**Contact Info**
_____	_____	_____
_____	_____	_____
_____	_____	_____
_____	_____	_____
_____	_____	_____

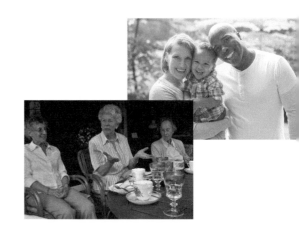

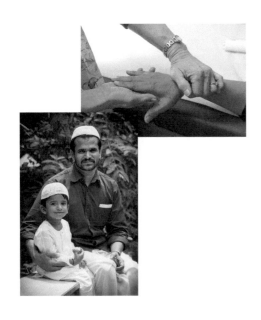

Appendix

Examples of Burdens and Values

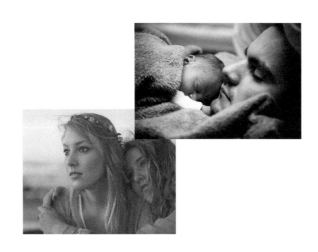

Examples of Burdens and Values

POSSIBLE DIFFICULTIES of TREATMENT or
THE WORKLOAD INVOLVED IN BEING A PATIENT
Sometimes, the inability to just be a person and not a patient any more

BURDENS OF TREATMENT - some *Examples* include:

- Visits to the doctor
- Stress
- Monitoring medication
- Physical responses, i.e. nausea, vomiting, etc.
- Medical tests
- Treatment convenience
- Scheduling flexibility
- Lifestyle impact
- Emotional / regimen distress
- Struggle with overall treatment
- Treatment management
- Lifestyle changes
- May not want to take pills or drink or eat

- Can't afford medication
- Trust that recommendations will work
- Monitoring vital signs
- Coming to all appointments
- Education level
- Literacy – ability to read and write
- Depression
- Pain
- Fatigue – tired of being sick – taking medication every day
- Social connectivity and supports
- Financial status

Any of these examples can affect capacity to do the work. The workload can simply exceed capacity to cope.

On top of feeling sick a lot, juggling family, work and social life takes so much time and effort that it can get to be too much to handle.

PERSONAL VALUES – for *Example* "I value_____"

- Hard work
- Independence
- Positive attitude
- Practicality
- Privacy
- Family closeness
- Make my own decisions
- Competitiveness
- Appearance
- Authority-control over activities
- Competition

- Physical work
- Power-having influence and the ability to act on it
- Knowledge
- Leadership
- Personal development
- Quality relationships
- Self-respect
- Order
- Serenity
- Self-reliance

My Values:

1. _____

2. _____

3. _____

4. _____

5. _____

My Burdens:

1. _____ 6. _____

2. _____ 7. _____

3. _____ 8. _____

4. _____ 9. _____

5. _____ 10._____

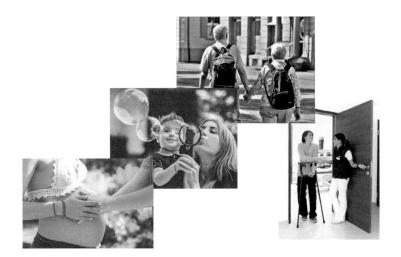

"*I cannot do everything but I can do something. I must not fail to do the something I can do.*"

~ Helen Keller

References

1. **O'Connor A, Wennberg JE, Legare F, Llewellyn-Thomas HA, Moulton BW, Sepucha KR, et al.** Toward the "tipping point": decision aids and informed patient choice. Health Aff. 2007;26(3):716–25.CrossRefGoogle Scholar

2. **Elwyn G, Coulter A, Laitner S, Walker E, Watson P, Thomson R.** Implementing shared decision making in the NHS. BMJ. 2010;341:c5146.PubMedCrossRefGoogle Scholar

3. Department of Health. Equity and excellence: liberating the NHS. London: 2010.Google Scholar

4. Senate and House of Representatives. Patient Protection and Affordable Care Act. HR 3590. Washington: 2010.Google Scholar

5. **Makoul G, Clayman ML.** An Integrative Model of Shared Decision Making in Medical Encounters. Patient Educ Couns. 2006;60:301–12.PubMedCrossRefGoogle Scholar

6. President's Commission. President's Commission for the Study of Ethical Problems in Medicine and Biomedical and Behavioral Research. Making Health Care Decisions. The Ethical and Legal Implications of Informed Consent in the Patient–Practitioner Relationship. Washington DC: 1982.Google Scholar

7. **Levenstein J.** The patient-centred general practice consultation. S Afr Fam Pract. 1984;5:276–82.Google Scholar

8. **Barry MJ, Edgman-Levitan S.** Shared decision making--pinnacle of patient-centered care. New Engl J Med. 2012;366(9):780–1. PubMedCrossRefGoogle Scholar

9. **Emanuel EJ, Emanuel LL.** Four models of the physician-patient relationship. JAMA. 1992;267:2221.PubMedCrossRefGoogle Scholar

10. **Charles C, Gafni A, Whelan T.** Shared decision-making in the medical encounter: what does it mean? (Or it takes at least two to tango). Soc Sci Med. 1997;44:681–92.PubMedCrossRefGoogle Scholar

11. **Towle A, Godolphin W.** Framework for teaching and learning informed shared decision making. BMJ. 1999;319:766–9. PubMedCrossRefGoogle Scholar

12. **Elwyn G, Edwards AG, Kinnersley P, Grol R.** Shared decision-making and the concept of equipoise: the competences of involving patients in healthcare choices. Br J Gen Pract. 2000;50(460):892–9.PubMedGoogle Scholar

13. **Ryan R, Deci E.** Self-determination theory and the facilitation of intrinsic motivation, social development, and well-being. Am Psychol. 2000;55(1):68–78.PubMedCrossRefGoogle Scholar

14. **Entwistle VA, Carter SM, Cribb A, McCaffery K.** Supporting patient autonomy: the importance of clinician-patient relationships. J Gen Intern Med. 2010;25(7):741–5.PubMedCrossRefGoogle Scholar

15. **Mackenzie C.** Relational autonomy, normative authority and perfectionism. J Soc Philos. 2008;39(4):512–33.CrossRefGoogle Scholar

16. **King J, Moulton B.** Rethinking Informed Consent: The Case for Shared Medical Decision-Making. Am J Law Med. 2006 Jan;32(4):429–501.PubMedGoogle Scholar

17. **Wear S.** Informed consent: Patient autonomy and clinician beneficence within health care. Washington DC: Georgetown Univ Pr; 1998.Google Scholar

18. **Zikmund-Fisher BJ, Couper MP, Singer E, Levin CA, Fowler FJ, Ziniel S, et al.** The DECISIONS study: a nationwide survey of United States adults regarding 9 common medical decisions. Med Decis Making. 30(5 Suppl):20 S–34S.Google Scholar

19. **Coulter A.** Do patients want a choice and does it work? BMJ. 2010;341:973–5.CrossRefGoogle Scholar

20. **Stewart M, Brown J, Weston W, McWinney I, McWilliam C, Freeman T.** Patient Centred Medicine: Transforming the Clinical Method. Thousand Oaks, CA: Sage Publications; 1995.Google Scholar

21. **Epstein RM, Alper BS, Quill TE.** Communicating Evidence for Participatory Decision Making. JAMA. 2004;291:2359–66. PubMedCrossRefGoogle Scholar

22. **Levinson W, Lesser CS, Epstein RM.** Developing physician communication skills for patient-centered care. Health affairs (Project Hope). 2010 Jul;29(7):1310–8.CrossRefGoogle Scholar

23. **Braddock CH, Fihn SD, Levinson W, Jonsen AR, Pearlman RA.** How doctors and patients discuss routine clinical decisions: informed decision making in the outpatient setting. 1997;12:339–45.PubMedGoogle Scholar

24. **Silverman J, Kurtz S, Draper J, Silverman J, Kurtz S, Draper J, et al.** Skills for communicating with patients. Abingdon: Radcliffe Medical Press; 1998.Google Scholar

25. **Stacey D, Bennett C, Barry M, Col N, Eden K, Holmes-Rovner, M Llewellyn-Thomas, H Lyddiatt A, et al.** Decision aids for people facing health treatment or screening decisions. Cochrane Database of Systematic Reviews. 2011;as well as(10):CD001431. Google Scholar

26. **Frosch D, Kaplan R.** Shared decision making in clinical medicine: past research and future directions. Am J Prev Med. 1999;17:285–94.PubMedCrossRefGoogle Scholar

27. **Schneider CE, CE S.** The practice of autonomy: patients, doctors, and medical decisions. New York: Oxford University Press; 1998. Google Scholar

28. **Gafni A, Charles C, Whelan T.** The physician-patient encounter: the physician as a perfect agent for the patient versus the informed decision-making model. Soc Sci Med. 1998;47(3):347–54.PubMedCrossRefGoogle Scholar

29. **O'Connor A, Bennett C, Stacey D, Barry M, Col N, Eden K, et al.** Decision aids for people facing health treatment or screening decisions. Cochrane Database of Systematic Reviews. 2009;Citation:(3):CD001431. doi: 10.1002/14651858.CD001431.

30. **Politi MC, Clark MA, Ombao H, Dizon D, Elwyn G.** Communicating uncertainty can lead to less decision satisfaction: a necessary cost of involving patients in shared decision making? Health Expectations [Internet]. 2011 Mar [cited 2011 Oct 4];14(1):84–91. Available from: doi:10.1111/j.1369-7625.2010.00626.x

31. **Quill T, Cassel C.** Nonabandonment: a central obligation for physicians. Ann Intern Med. 1995;122:368–74.PubMedGoogle Scholar

32. **Say R, Murtagh M, Thomson R.** Patients' preference for involvement in medical decision making: a narrative review. Patient Educ Counsel. 2006;60(2):102.CrossRefGoogle Scholar

33. **Epstein RM, Street RL.** Shared mind: communication, decision making, and autonomy in serious illness. Annals of Family Medicine. 9(5):454–61.Google Scholar

34. **Walter FM, Emery JD, Rogers M, Britten N.** Women's views of optimal risk communication and decision making in general practice consultations about the menopause and hormone replacement therapy. Patient Educ Counsel. 2004 May;53(2):121–8. CrossRefGoogle Scholar

35. **Epstein RM, Peters E.** Beyond information: exploring patients' preferences. JAMA. 2009;302(2):195–7.PubMedCrossRefGoogle Scholar

36. **Rapley T.** Distributed decision making: the anatomy of decisions-in-action. Sociol Health Illness. 2008;30(3):429–44. CrossRefGoogle Scholar

37. **Elwyn G, Miron-Shatz T.** Deliberation before determination: the definition and evaluation of good decision making. Health Expectations. 2009;13:139–47.PubMedCrossRefGoogle Scholar

38. **Elwyn G, Frosch D, Volandes AE, Edwards A, Montori VM.** Investing in Deliberation: A Definition and Classification of Decision Support Interventions for People Facing Difficult Health Decisions. Med Decis Making. 2010;30(6):701–11. PubMedCrossRefGoogle Scholar

39. **O'Connor A, Graham I, Visser A.** Implementing shared decision making in diverse health care systems: the role of patient decision aids. Patient Educ Counsel. 2005;57(3):247–9.CrossRefGoogle Scholar

40. **Elwyn G, Edwards A, Gwyn R, Grol R.** Towards a feasible model for shared decision making: focus group study with general practice registrars. BMJ. 1999;319(7212):753–6.PubMedCrossRefGoogle Scholar

41. **Hauer KE, Fernandez A, Teherani A, Boscardin CK, Saba GW.** Assessment of medical students' shared decision-making in standardized patient encounters. J Gen Intern Med. 2011;26(4):367–72.PubMedCrossRefGoogle Scholar

42. **Lloyd A, Joseph Williams N, Beasley A, Tomkinson A, Elwyn G.** Shared decision making in a multidisciplinary head and neck cancer team: a case study of developing Option Grids. International Journal of Person Centered Medicine. 2012;In Press. Google Scholar

43. **Braddock C, Edwards K, Hasenberg M, Laidley T, Levinson W.** Informed decision making in outpatient setting: time to get back to basics. JAMA. 1999;282:2313–20.PubMedCrossRefGoogle Scholar

44. **Elwyn G, Hutchings H, Edwards A, Rapport F, Wensing M, Cheung W-Y, et al.** The OPTION scale: measuring the extent that clinicians involve patients in decision-making tasks. Health Expectations. 2005;8(1):34–42.PubMedCrossRefGoogle Scholar

45. **Schiffrin D.** Discourse markers. Cambridge University Press; 1988.Google Scholar

46. **Edwards A, Elwyn G, Mulley A.** Explaining risks: turning numerical data into meaningful pictures. BMJ. 2002;324(7341):827–30. PubMedCrossRefGoogle Scholar

47. **Paling J.** Strategies to help patients understand risks. BMJ. 2003;327(7417):745–8.PubMedCrossRefGoogle Scholar

48. **Kurtz S, Silverman J.** The Calgary—Cambridge Referenced Observation Guides: an aid to defining the curriculum and organizing the teaching in communication training programmes. Med Educ. 1996;30(2):83–9.PubMedCrossRefGoogle Scholar

49. **Breslin M, Mullan RJ, Montori VM.** The design of a decision aid about diabetes medications for use during the consultation with patients with type 2 diabetes. Patient Educ Couns. 2008;73:465–72.PubMedCrossRefGoogle Scholar

50. **Whelan T, Levine M, Willan A, Gafni A, Sanders K, Mirsky D, et al.** Effect of a decision aid on knowledge and treatment decision making for breast cancer surgery: a randomized trial. JAMA. 2004;292(4):435.PubMedCrossRefGoogle Scholar

Copyright information

Printed in the United States
By Bookmasters